BEGINNER GUIDE TO NORDIC WALKING BENEFITS

Unlock The Ultimate Fitness Journey With Health Boosts, Weight Loss Strategies, And Cardio Workouts For Total Wellness And Joy

MALCOLM KASHTON

1

DISCLAIMER

This book contains information that is solely meant to be used for educational and informative reasons. This includes training regimens, game strategy, and fitness recommendations. Despite having taken every precaution to guarantee the correctness and completeness of the material provided, the author disclaims all express and implied warranties and representations regarding the content's suitability, timeliness, reliability, or accuracy for any purpose.

This book's content is not meant to be a replacement for expert medical advice, diagnosis, or care. When in doubt about a medical problem, never hesitate to consult your doctor or another trained healthcare professional. Never ignore medical advice from professionals or put off getting it because of something you've read in this book.

The material provided here and how you utilize it are not the responsibility of the author or publisher. You bear full responsibility for any reliance you make on the information contained in this book. The publisher and author disclaim all liability for any loss or damage resulting from using this book, including but not limited to indirect or consequential loss or damage, or any loss or damage from losing data or profits.

All references in this book to particular goods, services, or organizations are made for informative purposes only and do not imply endorsement or recommendation on the part of the publisher or author.

You acknowledge that there is no responsibility for any harm or injury that may arise from utilizing the material in this book, and that you will hold the author and publisher harmless by reading and using it. You alone are in charge of your own health and wellbeing, so you should apply any advice or suggestions from this book with caution and good judgment.

TABLE OF CONTENTS

ABOUT THE BOOK

"Nordic Walking Benefits" is a trustworthy resource that introduces readers to the practice of Nordic walking and offers a thorough analysis of all of its many benefits. Readers are introduced to the discipline in the introductory portion when the book lays the groundwork for comprehending its core ideas. The book is significant not just for revealing the historical foundations of Nordic walking but also for charting its development and rise to prominence.

The book on required gear and equipment is a crucial component of the book, offering readers guidance on selecting the best Nordic walking poles, shoes, and other accessories.

The section on mastering Nordic walking skills pays close attention to detail, emphasizing common faults and how to prevent them, ensuring that readers acquire a firm foundation in both fundamental form and advanced efficiency.

The book's examination of the various health advantages of Nordic walking is one of its most notable aspects. The book offers a wealth of information for anyone looking to improve their general well-being, from strengthening muscles and joints to improving cardiovascular health to managing weight effectively. It also explores the psychological and emotional advantages of Nordic walking, such as stress alleviation, mental clarity, and the social and communal aspects.

In addition, the book includes dedicated chapters that address the needs of particular demographic groups, including the elderly, people trying to lose weight, and those who use Nordic walking for injury prevention and rehabilitation. The practical value of the chapters on constructing Nordic walking routines and safety concerns is enhanced. These chapters provide readers with guidance on warm-up and cool-down exercises, workout development, and safe practice assurance.

In the end, "Nordic Walking Benefits" proves to be an invaluable resource for novices and experienced walkers alike. It is a helpful tool for people who want to include Nordic walking in their fitness regimens because it not only shares information on the history and methods of the exercise but also highlights its overall health advantages.

CHAPTER ONE

OVERVIEW OF NORDIC WALKING BENEFITS

GREETINGS FROM THE NORDIC WALKING WORLD

Welcome to the world of Nordic Walking, a full-body, dynamic exercise that combines the health benefits of walking with the assistance of specially designed poles. This distinctive and incredibly powerful workout has become more and more well-liked globally, providing devotees with a comprehensive approach to cardiovascular health, muscular engagement, and outdoor enjoyment. Let's explore the foundations of Nordic Walking as we begin this exploration to fully realize its potential to improve physical health and the outdoor experience as a whole.

Originally developed in Finland in the 1930s as a summer training technique for cross-country skiers, Nordic Walking is a unique type of exercise. It has developed into a stand-alone exercise routine that is suitable for individuals of all ages and physical levels throughout time. The use of specially crafted walking poles, which involve the upper body and turn a casual stroll into an intense workout, is what sets Nordic Walking apart. These poles, which are frequently height-adjustable, let users use a greater percentage of their muscles, increasing the activity's effectiveness and advantages over conventional walking.

RECOGNIZING THE FUNDAMENTALS OF NORDIC WALKING

Participants need to grasp the fundamentals of Nordic Walking to fully benefit from it. Nordic Walking, as opposed to casual walking, uses a diagonal arm and leg motion to produce a rhythmic and organic gait. In addition to moving the body forward, coordinating the swinging of the poles with each step works the shoulders, arms, and core, increasing calorie expenditure and enhancing muscle endurance. An easy stroll becomes a full-body workout as a result of this coordinated movement, which promotes a harmonious synergy between the upper and lower body.

Nordic walking poles are more than just accessories; they are essential to optimizing the health advantages of exercise. These poles, which are usually constructed from lightweight materials like carbon fiber or aluminum, have adjustable straps and ergonomic handles for the best possible comfort and support. By ensuring that the poles are positioned correctly, participants can walk with less pressure on their joints and more fluidity and efficiency.

Nordic walking is a flexible exercise that can be adjusted to different surfaces and levels of difficulty, making it appropriate for those with a range of fitness objectives. Nordic Walking can be customized to meet your unique goals, whether you're looking for a high-intensity workout to improve cardiovascular fitness or a low-impact activity to help with rehabilitation. Due to its accessibility and social interaction possibilities, it is a top option for people who want to improve their fitness regimen while taking use of nature.

We encourage you to experience the life-changing potential of Nordic Walking as we set off on our adventure. By comprehending its origins, accepting the distinctive method, and realizing the significance of specialty poles, participants can open a door to enhanced outdoor experiences, increased fitness, and better health. Now grab your poles, find your rhythm, and enjoy an exciting new experience in the world of Nordic Walking.

CHAPTER TWO

THE DEVELOPMENT AND HISTORY OF NORDIC WALKING

NORDIC WALKING'S HISTORICAL ORIGINS

The origins of Nordic Walking can be found in Finland in the early 1900s when it was developed as a winter training technique for cross-country skiers. The idea originated with Finnish ski instructors who used ski poles in their dryland training to keep their muscles engaged and their fitness levels intact. The foundation for Nordic Walking's development as a well-liked health and leisure activity was set by this early variation of the sport.

Nordic walking became well-known outside of its initial use as a skier training technique over time. The appeal of the sport grew as more people realized how special it was—full-body muscle activation combined with a cardiovascular workout. The idea of using poles to facilitate walking evolved into a core component of Nordic Walking, distinguishing it from traditional walking and transforming it into a unique form of exercise.

THE DEVELOPMENT OF NORDIC WALKING METHODS

Formal refining and the creation of defined procedures have been hallmarks of the development of Nordic Walking practices. Originally, the exercise was mostly walking with ski poles, but over time, participants and fitness professionals have improved the methods to get the most out of it.

To guarantee a smooth and effective walking experience, modern Nordic Walking techniques lay a strong emphasis on appropriate pole placement, arm movements, and coordinated strides. The purpose of the poles is to increase the overall cardiovascular workout, activate the upper body muscles, and offer stability. These improved methods have helped Nordic Walking become more and more popular, drawing in participants of all ages and fitness levels looking for a convenient and productive kind of exercise.

THE POPULARITY AND SPREAD OF NORDIC WALKING

Since its inception in Finland, Nordic Walking has seen a notable global expansion and increase in popularity. The sport became well-known worldwide in the 1990s as a full-body, low-impact workout that was appropriate for individuals of all ages and fitness levels.

Nordic walking's original association with winter sports gave way to applications in outdoor activities, rehabilitation regimens, and fitness regimens.

The allure of Nordic Walking is its adaptability; it may be done in a variety of places, including parks, trails, and cities. Its popularity among people looking for a fun and social way to do physical activity has been aided by its accessibility.

There are now numerous Nordic Walking organizations and groups that promote a feeling of camaraderie and a common love of this outdoor workout.

Fitness experts have been implementing Nordic Walking into their programs, and the wellness sector has embraced it in recent years. Nordic Walking's status as a popular and widely-used type of exercise has been cemented by the identification of its many health benefits, which include greater calorie burn, higher muscular strength, and improved cardiovascular fitness.

CHAPTER THREE

THE ESSENTIAL TOOLS AND DEVICES

THE BEST NORDIC WALKING POLE SELECTION

A comfortable and productive walking experience depends on choosing the right Nordic walking poles. Unlike standard hiking poles, these specialty poles are made to work the upper body and encourage a full-body workout. Material, length, and grip are important considerations when selecting Nordic walking poles.

The performance and longevity of the poles are largely dependent on the materials used. Carbon fiber poles are a popular option since they are lightweight and have good shock absorption. Conversely, aluminum poles provide both affordability and durability. For the best power transfer and a natural arm swing, the poles' length must be precisely adjusted based on your height.

The design of the grip is also important. Typically, ergonomic grips that offer a pleasant hold and effective power transfer are found on Nordic walking poles. Straps are included in certain grips to improve control and reduce hand fatigue. It's a good idea to test out various pole models to see which one best fits your walking style and preferences.

CHOOSING THE RIGHT SHOES FOR NORDIC WALKING

Selecting appropriate footwear is crucial for Nordic walking since it has a direct impact on comfort, stability, and overall effectiveness. Nordic walking requires shoes that assist the rolling motion from heel to toe and offer sufficient arch support. For comfort on longer hikes, shoes that are breathable and lightweight are ideal.

Seek out footwear with a naturally occurring range of motion and a flexible sole. The outsole should be able to manage many types of terrain with enough traction to give stability on both pavement and uneven ground. Make sure the shoes fit properly, with enough room for your toes without being too tight or too loose.

Hiking shoes with ankle support might be useful for anyone heading onto trails or uneven terrain. However, lighter athletic shoes might be more appropriate for paths that are kept up or in urban areas. To choose the best shoes for Nordic walking, you must try on various brands and styles and pay attention to how they feel when you walk.

ADDITIONAL CRUCIAL EQUIPMENT & ACCESSORIES

Apart from Nordic walking poles and appropriate footwear, a few additional necessary items and add-ons can improve the whole experience. To maintain your comfort level on walks of different intensities and to control body temperature, you need a base layer that is both breathable and moisture-wicking.

It's crucial to have a hydration system with you, like a hydration pack or water bottle, if you plan to go on longer hikes. Wearing sun protection, such as a hat, sunglasses, and sunscreen, is essential when engaging in outdoor activities to protect yourself from UV radiation.

You may carry necessities like extra layers of clothes, a first aid kit, and snacks in a well-fitting backpack. A fitness tracker or pedometer could be a good purchase to make goals and keep track of your progress. Finally, wear layers to adapt to changing weather conditions. If you intend to walk at night, remember to bring reflective clothing for enhanced protection.

CHAPTER FOUR

LEARNING THE TECHNIQUES OF NORDIC WALKING

FUNDAMENTAL FORM AND POSTURE OF NORDIC WALKING

Nordic walking, which involves walking with specially made poles, is a very accessible and effective full-body exercise. To get the most out of this exercise and reap the benefits, you must master the fundamental form and posture. Make sure your posture is relaxed and start by standing straight with your feet shoulder-width apart. Keep your elbows slightly bent and your body in an upright, natural position while holding the poles securely. Throughout the movement, maintain balance and stability by using your core muscles.

Compared to ordinary walking, Nordic walking has longer strides, which allows for more propulsion with each step. Plant the pole diagonally behind you as you swing your arms forward, then use your toes to lift off the ground. This encourages a full-body workout by using the muscles in your back, shoulders, and arms. To maintain a fluid stride, concentrate on moving in a smooth, rhythmic manner while coordinating the movement of your arms and legs.

MORE COMPLEX METHODS FOR EFFECTIVENESS

If you want to improve the effectiveness of your Nordic walking, you should think about using more sophisticated techniques that make use of the poles to generate more force and endurance. The double-poling method is one such technique in which the body is propelled forward by simultaneously using both poles.

This increases upper body engagement, escalating the intensity of the activity and enhancing cardiovascular fitness. Gaining proficiency in both uphill and downhill walking with poles will further strengthen and challenge your muscles.

Changing up the tempo and intensity of your Nordic walking practice is another sophisticated approach. Include quick walking intervals or brief jogging spurts, all while using the poles correctly. In addition to increasing your heart rate, this gives your exercise regimen more variety.

To maximize efficiency and effectiveness, keep in mind to experiment with these advanced techniques while maintaining a dynamic posture and fluid motion.

TYPICAL ERRORS AND HOW TO PREVENT THEM

Even while Nordic walking seems easy, there are a few typical faults that might reduce its benefits and enjoyment. Grasping the poles too tightly is a common mistake that causes needless strain on the hands and arms. To prevent this, keep your hands loosely gripping the handles so that your walking motion can be pleasant and natural.

Another frequent error is placing the pole incorrectly. With every step, make sure the poles are positioned diagonally behind you to give you the support and momentum you need. Refrain from hunching your shoulders or bending forward too much since this might put a strain on your back and neck. Rather, concentrate on keeping your body in an erect position, using your core, and letting the poles help you distribute your weight evenly.

Skipping appropriate warm-up and cool-down exercises is a mistake that can cause pain and even injury. Make flexibility and stretching exercises your priority to warm up your muscles for Nordic walking and avoid soreness afterward. Through correcting these common faults and practicing safe practices, you can become an expert Nordic walker and enjoy all of the physical and mental health benefits it offers.

CHAPTER FIVE

NORDIC WALKING'S HEALTH BENEFITS

ENHANCEMENT OF CARDIOVASCULAR HEALTH

Nordic walking has several prominent physical benefits, one of which is its beneficial effects on cardiovascular health. With the use of specially made poles, this low-impact, cardiovascular workout works both the upper and lower body. People's heart rates rise as they walk with rhythmic arm motions, which improve blood circulation. This improved circulation aids in the elimination of waste materials from the body as well as the more effective delivery of nutrients and oxygen throughout it.

Cardiovascular fitness gains have been linked to regular Nordic walking participation. Large muscle groups are activated by the combination of arm and leg motions, which increases cardiac workload.

The heart muscle is strengthened, its pumping efficiency is improved, and it adds to overall cardiovascular endurance when the strain is raised. Furthermore, it has been demonstrated that Nordic walking lowers blood pressure and promotes a healthier cardiovascular system by lowering the risk of hypertension.

BUILDING UP JOINTS AND MUSCLES

Nordic walking is unique as a full-body exercise because it works a variety of joints and muscle groups. The use of poles in Nordic walking engages the muscles in the arms, shoulders, and back, in contrast to regular walking, which places more emphasis on the lower body. In addition to increasing upper body strength, the constant pushing and pulling motion of the poles improves total muscular tone.

Nordic walking also offers a low-impact substitute for people with joint problems. By distributing the force of each stride throughout the whole body, the usage of poles lessens the strain on the ankles, hips, and knees.

Because of this, it's a good workout for people who want to build their muscles and joints without putting themselves through the high-impact strain that comes with things like running. Nordic walking can thus be an important part of recovery regimens for people recuperating from joint replacements or injuries.

LOSING WEIGHT AND BURNING CALORIES

Nordic walking is a useful strategy for burning calories and controlling weight. The activity's total energy expenditure is increased when walking quickly and using muscles in both the upper and lower bodies. When paired with a healthy diet, this increased caloric expenditure can help with weight loss or maintenance.

Moreover, Nordic walking offers a fun and sustainable type of exercise, increasing the likelihood that people will stick to a regular fitness schedule. This activity's adaptability makes it suitable for a wide range of fitness levels by letting participants adjust the intensity of their workout. It thus becomes an important part of comprehensive weight-management plans that enhance general well-being and physical activity.

CHAPTER SIX
EMOTIONAL AND MENTAL HEALTH
RELAXATION AND STRESS REDUCTION

Reducing stress and relaxing are essential for maintaining a balanced and healthy lifestyle when it comes to mental and emotional well-being. Stress, which is frequently seen as an inevitable part of contemporary life, can be harmful to one's physical and emotional well-being. Putting into practice practical stress-reduction strategies is essential for preserving general well-being. It has been demonstrated that techniques including progressive muscular relaxation, deep breathing, and mindfulness meditation reduce stress by encouraging serenity and relaxation. These methods support long-term emotional resilience in addition to helping to manage the short-term impacts of stress.

Furthermore, pursuing happy and fulfilling pursuits might serve as effective stress relievers.

Engaging in artistic endeavors, hobbies, or time spent in nature can all be beneficial ways to decompress. Achieving and preserving mental equilibrium depends on identifying and resolving stressors, whether they are interpersonal, work-related, or personal. Adopting a holistic strategy that integrates techniques for mental and physical well-being can greatly reduce stress, which in turn promotes a resilient and upbeat outlook.

NORDIC WALKING AND EMOTIONAL RESOLVE

Nordic walking, a type of walking that uses specially made poles, is becoming more and more popular since it improves mental clarity in addition to physical health. This low-impact workout improves cardiovascular health and works a variety of muscle groups, which enhances general well-being. Nordic walking has been linked to improved mental focus and cognitive function in addition to its physical benefits.

Nordic walking's deliberate and rhythmic motions, along with the outdoor activities' tendency to foster a sense of connection to nature, foster an atmosphere that is favorable to mental clarity. Engaging in physical activity and spending time outdoors have been associated with happier and less anxious sentiments. When done in groups, the social component of Nordic walking also contributes to mental well-being by fostering a sense of success and camaraderie. Essentially, Nordic walking is a holistic exercise that supports the mind and body in addition to its physical advantages.

BENEFITS TO THE COMMUNITY AND SOCIETY

Since social interactions are fundamental to human nature, the value of social ties for mental and emotional health cannot be emphasized. Emotional support and a sense of belonging are greatly enhanced by social interaction and community involvement. A strong social network has been associated with reduced stress, anxiety, and depression rates, demonstrating the significant influence of social networks on mental health.

Finding purpose and fulfillment can come from volunteering, taking part in community events, or just spending time with loved ones. A support network is formed via the sharing of experiences and the exchange of emotional support, which serves as a buffer against life's adversities. A sense of identification and belonging is also fostered by community involvement, which enhances mental health.

The field of mental and emotional well-being is greatly influenced by a variety of factors, including stress management and relaxation techniques, the mental clarity that comes from exercises like Nordic walking, and the social and communal advantages of human interaction. Taking a comprehensive approach that incorporates these ideas can help you live a more fulfilling, resilient, and balanced life.

CHAPTER SEVEN

NORDIC WALKING FOR PARTICULAR GROUPS

SENIORS WHO LIKE NORDIC WALKING

Nordic walking has grown in popularity as a low-impact, full-body workout that is good for people of all ages. Seniors, in particular, can get a lot of benefits from this type of exercise. Walking poles with unique designs improve stability and lessen joint stress, making it a viable form of exercise for senior citizens. Nordic walking has been shown to improve cardiovascular fitness, strengthen muscles, and improve balance in seniors. These benefits all contribute to increased mobility and a lower risk of falls.

The versatility of Nordic walking to suit varying levels of fitness is a major benefit for senior citizens. Seniors can easily modify the activity's intensity to customize their workouts to meet their unique demands and physical capabilities.

Additionally, the social component of Nordic walking can be advantageous for senior citizens, offering chances for engagement in groups and social interactions that promote well-being and a sense of community.

WALKING NORDIC STYLE TO REDUCE WEIGHT

Nordic walking is a weight loss or weight management technique that is both effective and enjoyable to exercise. Compared to conventional walking, the use of walking poles increases total energy expenditure by using the upper body muscles. When paired with a balanced diet, this contributes to weight loss by resulting in a more effective burn of calories.

Nordic walking is a great aerobic activity that improves cardiovascular health and promotes fat burning because of its rhythmic and repeated nature. Furthermore, each stride's activation of the core muscles contributes to the abdominal region's strengthening. Because Nordic walking is accessible to people of all fitness levels, it's a good option for people who are just starting to lose weight or are searching for a long-term, sustainable workout regimen.

NORDIC WALKING AS A REHAB AND INJURY PREVENTION METHOD

Because Nordic walking is low-impact and uses poles to disperse the burden over the entire body, it has been acknowledged as an effective method for injury prevention and recovery.

Nordic walking offers a means of physical activity without overstressing joints and muscles for people recuperating from injuries or managing long-term ailments.

Nordic walking can help restore normal muscle function and gait patterns because of its controlled and symmetrical motions, which makes it an appropriate rehabilitation activity for a variety of musculoskeletal conditions.

Walking poles can help with balance maintenance and lower the chance of falls while recovering.

 Enhancing total body coordination and fortifying the core muscles help prevent injuries. Nordic walking supports good posture and stability, which helps people develop a foundation of strength that can lower their risk of injury from everyday activities. All things considered, Nordic walking proves to be a flexible, all-inclusive exercise that has numerous advantages for both injury prevention and rehabilitation.

CHAPTER EIGHT

ESTABLISHING NORDIC WALKING SCHEDULES

CREATING EFFECTIVE WARM-UP AND COOL-DOWN EXERCISES

A well-thought-out warm-up and cool-down is an essential part of any Nordic walking program. Warm-up activities raise heart rate and improve blood flow to muscles, readying the body for the physical activity that lies ahead. Dynamic stretches that work both the upper and lower body are perfect for Nordic walking. During an exercise, improved range of motion is encouraged by performing arm circles, leg swings, and torso twists to help loosen up muscles and joints. To prime the cardiovascular system for the following workout, gradually raise the intensity.

To prevent dizziness or pain, cool-down activities are equally crucial in gradually restoring the body's temperature and pulse rate to normal. Increasing flexibility and lowering soreness in the muscles can be achieved by incorporating static stretches that focus on the main muscle groups engaged in Nordic walking.

An emphasis on the calves, hips, shoulders, and arms helps improve joint mobility and postural alignment. Individual fitness levels should be taken into account when designing warm-up and cool-down exercises. This will help participants recover from their workout and ensure they are ready for the main Nordic walking session.

CREATING A DIVERSITY OF NORDIC WALKING WORKOUTS

Adding interest and diversity to a routine helps to keep participants motivated and interested. A popular method is interval training, which alternates between slower recovery intervals and intervals of vigorous walking. This works a variety of muscle groups and improves cardiovascular fitness.

Including both uphill and downhill terrain intensifies the workout by focusing on the lower body and increasing total strength.

For novices, it's important to concentrate on developing good form and escalating duration and intensity gradually. Resistance training combined with Nordic walking poles can offer an increased challenge as participants develop, better using the muscles in the upper body. For individuals who are looking for endurance benefits, long-distance Nordic walking sessions can also be included. The secret is to customize exercises to meet personal fitness objectives and levels to create a fun and challenging environment.

INCLUDING NORDIC WALKING IN YOUR EXERCISE PROGRAM

Including Nordic walking in your workout program requires that you match the exercise to your objectives and preferences. Important first stages include determining one's current level of fitness, taking into account any pre-existing medical issues, and setting reasonable goals. Nordic walking is an accessible option for people of all ages because it can be tailored to different fitness levels.

Incorporating Nordic walking into an overall fitness plan requires scheduling regular sessions throughout the week. A well-rounded fitness program is produced by incorporating Nordic walking with other types of exercise, such as strength training or flexibility exercises. Furthermore, getting help from a qualified instructor or taking part in group Nordic walking sessions can boost motivation and foster a sense of community.

The secret to successfully implementing Nordic walking into a fitness regimen is customization, slow growth, and an all-encompassing strategy that takes mental and physical health into account. Nordic walking may make a big difference in your overall fitness and health, whether you use it as your main workout or as a supplement.

CHAPTER NINE

SAFETY POINTS TO REMEMBER

GUIDELINES FOR NORDIC WALKING SAFETY

There are several health advantages to Nordic walking, a full-body exercise that involves walking with specially-made poles. It is imperative to guarantee safety throughout this exercise, nevertheless. First and foremost, it's critical to employ the appropriate tools. Select poles with comfortable grips and the appropriate height. It's also essential to have appropriate footwear to avoid falls and slides.

A key factor in avoiding injuries during Nordic walking is using proper technique. Keep your shoulders back, your core tight, and your arms swing naturally. To give your body time to adjust, start with shorter sessions and progressively increase the intensity. To minimize the danger of strains or sprains, warm-up activities are crucial for preparing muscles and joints for the activity.

When Nordic walking, being aware of your surroundings is crucial for safety. Select well-kept paths, use caution on uneven terrain, and keep an eye out for impediments such as rocks or roots. Pay attention to your surroundings, especially if you're strolling close to a car. When strolling in groups, make eye contact with other pedestrians to prevent accidents and guarantee a comfortable stroll.

TYPICAL ACCIDENTS AND HOW TO AVOID THEM

Even though Nordic walking has many advantages, injuries can still happen if the right safety measures are not followed. Shin splints are one common injury that is frequently brought on by overuse or incorrect technique.

Make sure your poles are the right length and refrain from overstriding to prevent shin injuries. Walk for longer periods and with increasing intensity gradually to give your body time to adjust.

Blisters are another common problem that arises from the friction that occurs between your skin and the equipment. Blisters can be avoided by wearing socks that wick away moisture and shoes that fit correctly. Make sure you regularly inspect your equipment for signs of wear and tear because defective equipment can lead to accidents.

Pushing yourself too hard without the right preparation might lead to strains in your muscles and damage to your joints. Stretching exercises for the main muscle groups involved in Nordic walking should be incorporated into your warm-up before each session. By adding variation to your fitness regimen, cross-training with other activities can also help prevent overuse problems.

CLIMATE AND SAFETY IN THE ENVIRONMENT

The safety of Nordic walking can be greatly impacted by weather and environmental factors. In hot weather, avoid walking during the hottest hours of the day and drink plenty of water. Wear lightweight clothing, a hat, and sunscreen for the weather. Wear layers of clothing in chilly weather to stay warm and prevent frostbite on your extremities.

Being aware of the environment is essential for safety. Respect wildlife and refrain from altering their natural habitats. Use poles for stability and adapt your technique to the conditions while you're in places with different terrain. When it's raining or snowing, use caution on slick surfaces and think about utilizing poles with rubber tips for increased traction.

Before leaving, always check the weather prediction, and be ready for any unforeseen changes. Keep emergency supplies like a first aid kit, a cell phone that has been charged, and a map with you. Tell someone about your plans to go walking, particularly if you're going somewhere distant or less crowded, to make sure that safety comes first.

CHAPTER TEN

INVESTIGATING NORDIC WALKING PATHS

LOCATING THE GREATEST PATHS FOR NORDIC WALKING

Discovering Nordic walking trails means venturing into a realm where the natural world and exercise coexist in harmony. Finding the greatest Nordic walking routes requires giving careful thought to several aspects, including the topography, degree of difficulty, and scenic beauty of each path's surroundings. Nordic walking aficionados, whether they are novices seeking easy routes or seasoned walkers seeking more difficult terrain, frequently hunt for trails that suit their ability levels. To find these undiscovered treasures and guarantee an enjoyable and rewarding Nordic walking experience, local trail guides, internet resources, and community recommendations become invaluable tools.

GETTING IN TOUCH WITH THE OUTDOORS AND NATURE

The chance to establish a deep connection with nature is one of the main draws of Nordic walking routes. Nordic walking's rhythmic motion heightens the sensory experience as participants make their way through verdant forests, peaceful meadows, or scenic beaches. In addition to offering a full-body workout, moving forward with customized poles lets people take in the sights, sounds, and smells of the surrounding environment. Being in nature has long been known to have therapeutic effects, including increasing mental health and a sense of tranquility, which is enhanced by Nordic walking expeditions.

TRAVELING WITH NORDIC WALKING: AN ADVENTURE

Walking on the Nordic Trail has become a popular niche in the larger outdoor activity market. Travelers from all over the world are drawn to locations that provide outstanding Nordic walking paths together with a comprehensive experience that incorporates local charm and cultural immersion. Beyond the physical features of Nordic walking, these walking tours offer a diverse trip through historical sites, cultural hubs, and picturesque panoramas. Communities that welcome Nordic walking tourism see it as a chance to highlight their distinctive cultural legacy and unspoiled natural beauty, promoting a mutually beneficial partnership between outdoor enthusiasts and local businesses.

Discovering Nordic walking trails requires a careful search for paths that accommodate different tastes and skill levels. These pathways offer a venue for deeply and personally connecting with nature, promoting both physical and mental well-being.